I0412603

"Black Jack"
to Prevent a Surgery Setback

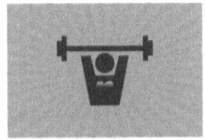

A guide to achieving wellness
before, during, and after a surgical experience!

Carpe Diem
Seize the day—every day!

Stacey Alexis Karseras, LPN

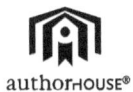

authorHOUSE®

AuthorHouse™
1663 Liberty Drive
Bloomington, IN 47403
www.authorhouse.com
Phone: 1-800-839-8640

© 2012 Stacey Alexis Karseras LPN. All rights reserved.
 www.blackjacktolosefat.info

No part of this book may be reproduced, stored in a retrieval system, or
transmitted by any means without the written permission of the author.

Published by AuthorHouse 5/14/2012

ISBN: 978-1-4685-9521-5 (e)
ISBN: 978-1-4685-9523-9 (sc)

Library of Congress Control Number: 2012907795

Any people depicted in stock imagery provided by Thinkstock are models,
and such images are being used for illustrative purposes only.
Certain stock imagery © Thinkstock.

This book is printed on acid-free paper.

Because of the dynamic nature of the Internet, any web addresses or links contained in
this book may have changed since publication and may no longer be valid. The views
expressed in this work are solely those of the author and do not necessarily reflect the
views of the publisher, and the publisher hereby disclaims any responsibility for them.

Concorde Career Center: CNA
School of Fitness and Nutrition Phoenix, Az certification in fitness and nutrition
Erwin Technical Center School of Nursing: LPN

Preface

I would like to begin by thanking anyone who has purchased any of my *"Black Jack"* books. In the course of speaking to a number of patients, I learned that most were uneducated about the condition of their own health and the risks before, during, and after a surgical procedure.

Most of them are seeking guidance but just don't know whether or in what way their health is already compromised by a health condition. I promote better health by educating others with information I have observed in the last twenty-five years working in health care. *"Black Jack"* is the focus, which has nothing to do with the card game; the term suggests that none of us should gamble with our livelihood and why it is important to become or remain healthy, lose or prevent fat, get your health back, and prevent a surgery setback.

I've observed family members, friends, and patients who have had surgery. No two surgeries are the same because everyone has a different lifestyle that can affect the outcome or prognosis. Preparation and attention to detail is the responsibility of both health care personnel and the patient.

Contents

Introduction

Surgery is an invasive procedure because it involves cutting through layers of skin. The thought of having surgery is scary to most people. The decision to have surgery, even if it is medically necessary to prolong life, is sometimes a difficult one. Every patient has rights and the choice to create an advance directive giving specific instructions to others in regard to life saving measures. You may also use an advance directive to appoint another person to make medical or financial decisions on your behalf.

Before a surgical procedure, you must sign many consent forms, including those pertaining to the risks of surgery, anesthetics, and consent to treat. Risk factors vary with each patient resulting from the type of procedure to be performed, the length of the surgery, the anesthetic to be given, bleeding, and the patient's lifestyle, habits, age, medical history, and body weight. Everyone has risks. If a patient withholds information regarding medical or substance abuse during the pre-op process, the risk for complications may increase. An anesthesiologist watches for red flags that require appropriate prevention or preparation to decrease a patient's risk for complications prior to, during, or after a procedure. It is possible for a surgery to be cancelled on its scheduled day if the patient has withheld information.

Health care employees have the common goal of helping to maintain the quality of life and well-being of other persons, but each patient has responsibilities, too.

Advance Directives

Advance directives include many types of legal documentation regarding health and financial decisions.

A *living will* (LW) is enforced if an individual is unable to make medical decisions.

A *health care surrogate* (HCS) appoints another person to make health care decisions on someone else's behalf.

A *power of attorney* (POA) appoints another person to make legal decisions on someone else's behalf.

A *do not resuscitate* (DNR) states an individual's wishes regarding life saving measures in case of an emergency.

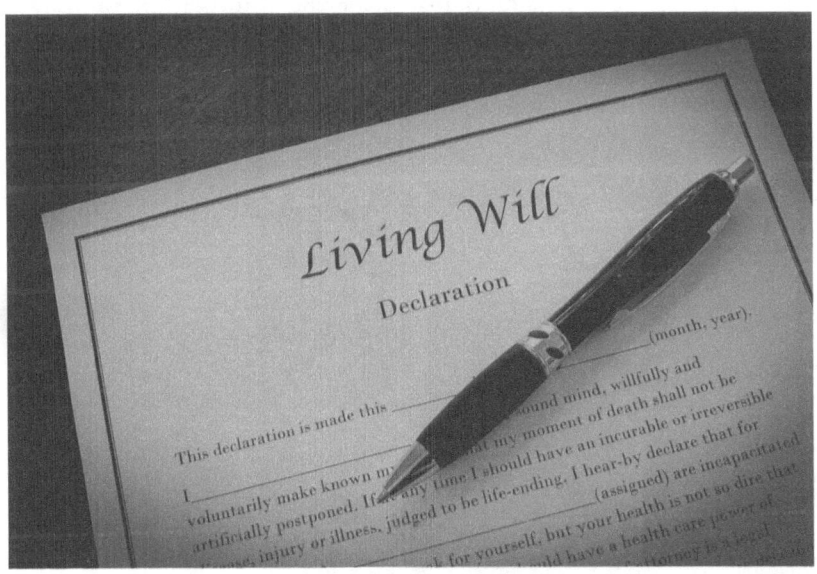

Consent Forms

Have you ever wondered why the use of small print is so common, especially on legal documents? This information is usually the most important and is often overlooked. It usually takes a few more minutes to read and may be difficult to understand but might include details a salesman hopes a customer will just skim over. These documents can be used in a court of law, so the time to ask questions is before signing. It is everyone's right to understand any document prior to signing it, so take the time to read each document thoroughly before signing.

No question is a stupid question!

Before any procedure, you may have several interviews with medical personnel to see how good of a candidate you are for the procedure in question. Each patient should read over the information thoroughly before scheduling a procedure and ask plenty of questions about anything unclear.

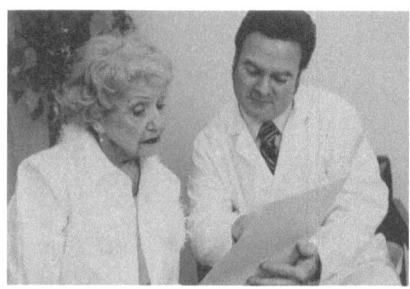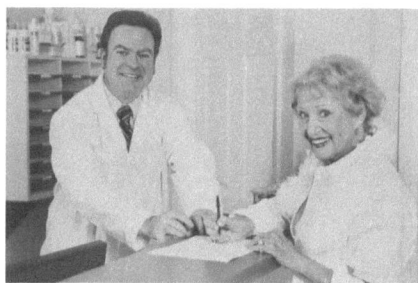

Necessary Versus Elective Surgery

If you have an accident or medical emergency, surgery may be the only option that will allow you to maintain your quality of life. You may not have time to make the decision on your own or to seek a second opinion. A medical professional's goal is to preserve a patient's quality of life unless otherwise instructed by an advanced directive. If you are considering a surgery that is not a medical emergency but may increase your quality of life, then you should consider the risks before scheduling the procedure, meet with the surgeon, and ask questions regarding pre-op, surgery, post-op, and your individual prognosis. A surgeon may have reservations or refuse to perform surgery on someone because of a person's lifestyle or habits, for example, if the patient uses nicotine, alcohol, or recreational drugs.

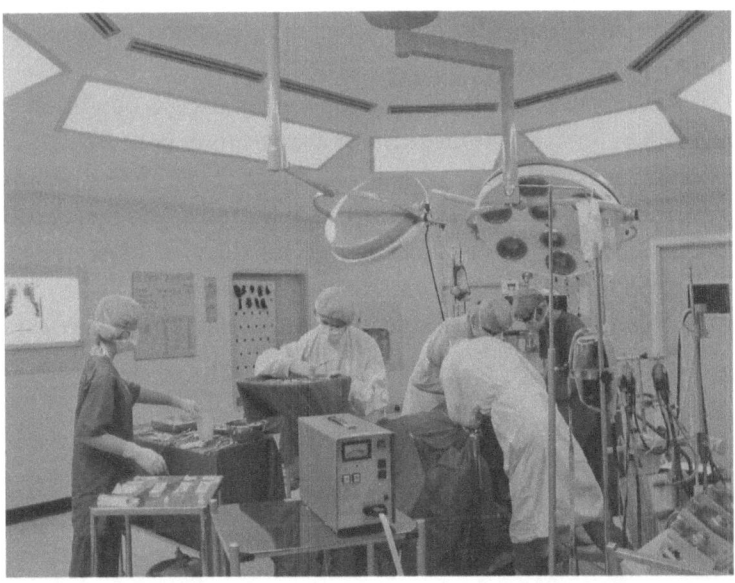

Medical History

A patient's *medical history* tells a story or paints a picture for a healthcare professional. Many patients are uneducated in regard to their own health, but this information is very important and may determine the prognosis before a procedure is ever performed. Undisclosed information may place a patient at an increased risk for complications. Anytime you have an acute (onetime) or chronic (occurring more than once) illness, it becomes part of your medical history. Sometimes, a procedure is cancelled on the day it is scheduled because a patient forgot to mention pertinent information during the preoperative process, such as substance abuse. I've learned that the majority of cardiac patients are unaware that high blood pressure (the silent killer) and elevated cholesterol levels are both heart problems.

An anesthesiologist reviews a patient's medical history prior to the date of service to enable proper facility placement, prevention, and preparation appropriate for each case.

A physician can prescribe medication for a particular condition, but if the patient does not take the medicine or change his or her current lifestyle, the condition is usually still present and most of the time unmanaged. Medication is not a cure to a problem and may even create more problems or secondary conditions resulting from risks for allergies, adverse reactions, and side effects. The more information a patient is able to divulge, the better the chance medical personnel have to provide appropriate care.

Surgical History

After a patient has an invasive procedure, it becomes part of the patient's medical history. If someone is experiencing a health problem and decides to seek a physician's recommendation for treatment, the least invasive action is usually initiated before surgery is performed. This may include changes in lifestyle, habits, rehabilitation, or pain management. Anyone with uncontrolled health problems increases his risks with surgery. Many surgeons will not perform surgery if the patient does not comply with preoperative instructions prior to scheduling a procedure or if that person's lifestyle or habits, such as nicotine, alcohol, and drug abuse, cause risks for additional complications that are too high. A surgeon always seeks a positive outcome or prognosis, and most do not like to see their patients experience complications or to perform multiple surgeries made necessary by complications. It is important to always check if the physician is board certified for the procedure in question. In many circumstances a person's history may cause a surgeon to hesitate before scheduling the procedure, and the surgeon will make the final decision to treat or perform it.

Anesthetics

An *anesthetic* is an agent used for numbing. The route an anesthetic is administered can vary. Several factors are used to determine the best route for each patient, such as age, medical history, the type or length of surgery, and bleeding risk. An anesthesiologist treats each patient individually. A positive outcome with the fewest complications is the primary goal of every procedure.

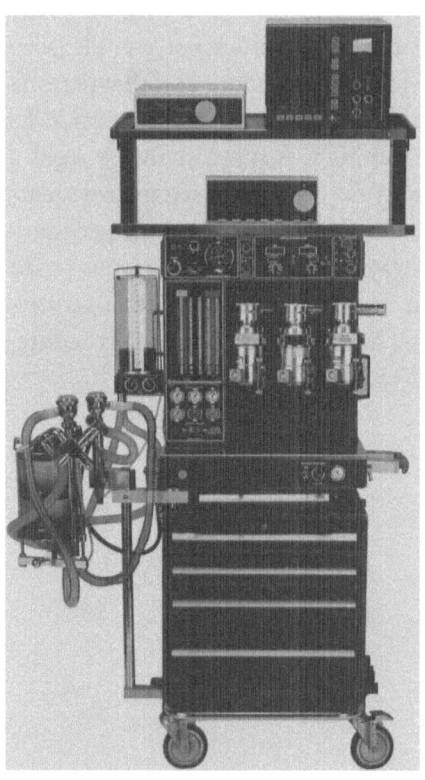

The anesthesiologist will decide the best route and will provide instructions to decrease complications before and after administering the anesthetic. Three types of administration are local, regional, and general. Local and regional anesthetics leave the patient conscious during sedation. General anesthetics may be used with procedures that have an increased risk for bleeding, but a person's medical history may be the deciding factor because of the additional risk for complications. Medicine is sometimes given in doses computed by a patient's weight. Body fat percentage may alter a person's metabolism and the amount of anesthetic given.

The best prevention for preparation is to alert medical personnel if you or any of your blood relatives have ever had a reaction of any type from an anesthetic.

Risks of Anesthetics

Anyone who receives an anesthetic is at risk for complications. Reactions may include allergic or other adverse side effects. A patient who has received an anesthetic before is not immune to these risks, and even the healthiest people are at risk for complications. A few allergic reactions are hives, itching, and anaphylaxis (swelling of the tongue and throat). Common side effects are nausea, vomiting, headache, crying, anxiety, and anger. Other complications are early awakening, delayed awakening, unstable vital signs, decreased oxygen saturation levels, malignant hyperthermia (high temperature), and cardiac arrest. A patient with multiple health problems has an increased risk if the medical problems are not managed with lifestyle or medication or if the patient has secondary conditions from medication. A patient with this type of history may require surgery to be scheduled at a hospital in case of complications, because additional support systems are already in place. A person's lifestyle and habits will also increase the risk for complications, especially nicotine, alcohol, and drug abuse. Prevention is the key to reducing such risks, and disclosing this information prior to surgery is very important in order to maintain quality of life before, during, and after surgery.

Anesthetic History

Prior to a procedure, a patient will be interviewed by a series of medical personnel to answer questions regarding that person's health history, lifestyle, and habits. Every time an anesthetic is received, the same risks apply and can reoccur, so any information disclosed during the preoperative process will educate personnel how to provide proper prevention and preparation necessary to decrease the risks. If medical professionals are aware of health problems prior to scheduling surgery, then facility placement, prevention and preparation can be initiated. Problems for them to be aware of include any personal or family history of any symptoms during and after receiving an anesthetic.

Immune System

The *immune system* is our defense against illness and diseases that include cancer. Several factors can compromise this system. Lifestyle, health, and habits can predispose a person for resistance to the common cold or flu. Both are viral infections. The length of time a person may have symptoms varies and depends on individual immunity, prevention, and treatment of symptoms. Consistent nourishment choices rich in nutrients and antioxidants, such as citrus fruit, berries, dark chocolate, vegetables, or shellfish, may improve immunity. Resistance training is another building block for better long-term health and will reduce inflammation and pain. *"Black Jack"* 21 and the *(Advanced Version)* are programs included in my books, *"Black Jack"* to lose fat and *"Black Jack"* to get your health back. Two full body resistance training programs, I recommend three times a week in the comfort of your own space. Both circuits can take as little as thirty minutes.

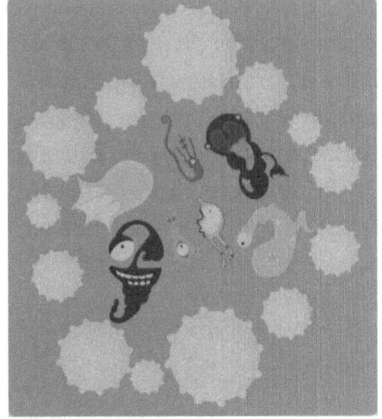

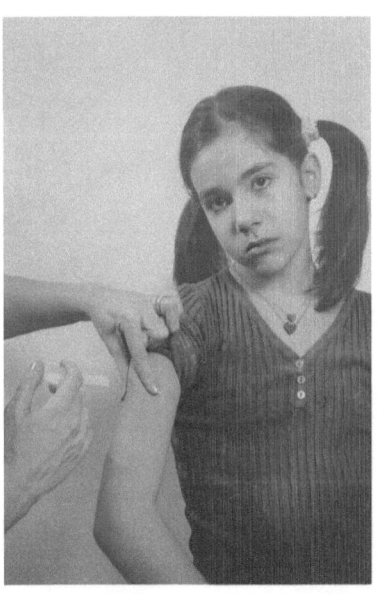

Infection

An *infection* can be local or systemic. A local infection can usually be seen. A fever may be present in either kind. Other symptoms may include pain, redness, drainage, odor, nausea, vomiting, chills, and lethargy. Infection can invade cells, tissues, bone, and blood, so it is very important to address symptoms immediately. Infection can start with the bacteria on the surface of the skin but can invade deeper tissue, organs, bone, and blood very fast. If the infection reaches the blood stream, septic shock and death can occur.

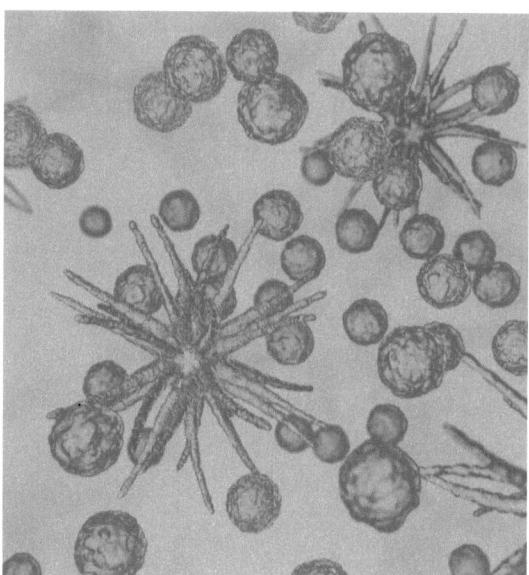

A person's lifestyle, habits, and history of antibiotic usage sometimes make it more difficult to kill certain bacteria. Fighting an infection that lasts for years may affect a person's quality of life and state of mind.

Physical Fitness

Lack of mobility equals lack of motility. Sometimes as we get older, our level of activity changes. Even though fitness is an important factor to maintaining mobility, everyone is susceptible to injuries from repetitive movements, overuse, or weak muscles and bones. Several activities can place added pressure on the joints, muscles, and bones, such as jogging, running, and tennis. Consistent resistance training is the best type of exercise to increase lean muscle mass, produce vitamins and minerals naturally, improve calcium levels and bone strength, prevent or decrease fat, allow a person to be remain active and agile, and maintain muscle tone. A strong core (between the neck and waist) will support the body. Those who participate in any activity for recreation or sport can benefit from any resistance training program, such as *"Black Jack" 21* and anyone over the age of four can resistance train with proper supervision, so the

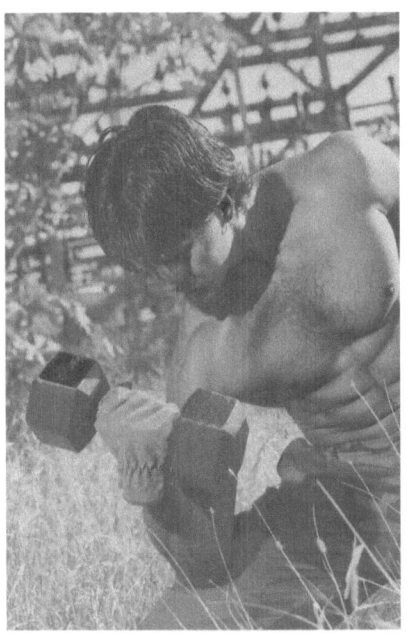

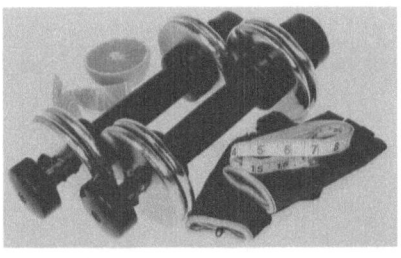

whole family can exercise together. (Always seek medical advice prior to beginning any fitness or nutrition program.) Allow the body to react to the changes that this type of exercise provides—especially the cardiovascular system, because it is the key to heart health and staying alive. High blood pressure (the silent killer), being the most common heart problem, is often overlooked. But resistance training helps to lower blood pressure, pain, cravings, and increase oxygen levels for more cardiovascular health benefits, and it helps to stabilize hormones, metabolism, and mood. These types of exercises will also lower blood sugar levels and provide a natural, good feeling that will keep you coming back for more.

Scar Tissue and Adhesions

Our skin is the protective barrier between the elements and our internal organs. A break in this barrier can cause infection and other problems. Cuts, abrasions, and first-degree burns are superficial wounds and usually heal without difficulty or minor scarring. Breaks in the skin resulting from trauma, incisions, or surgery are deeper than the first layer of skin and involve underlying tissue that is more difficult to heal because of the lack of blood flow necessary for new tissue growth. The tissue is replaced with a protein called collagen. Scar tissue can adhere to internal organs and cause other complications, even additional surgeries. Scars appear differently on each patient, the result of many factors, including infection, other complications, ethnicity, and the tendency to develop keloid. Wound care will require treatments to promote healing. A person's lifestyle or habits can affect this process. Anytime the immune system is compromised, the risk for complications increases. Over time, further treatments and surgeries may be necessary, thus impairing a person's quality of life or state of mind.

Wound Dehiscence

Wound dehiscence (splitting open) at the incision site is a risk that is present with most surgical procedures. The incision may open, exposing tissue and causing bleeding or hemorrhage. It can become very dangerous. Several factors increase the risk, such as a person's lifestyle and habits, placement of the sutures, and patient responsibility. Following the doctor's orders, wound care treatments and proper health will increase the chance for a more positive prognosis. If the sutures are placed in an area of high mobility, for example, the abdomen, elbow, or knee, then the chance for a wound to dehisce is greater, and immobility may be required to prevent this from occurring. This is usually caused by a patient trying to do too much too soon. Another cause is an obese patient putting additional pressure on the incision site. Proper nutrition, health, and lifestyle are required for the best outcome. Patients have a huge responsibility in terms of their prognosis. Surgical error is rarely the cause of most complications, but it does occur.

Incisional Hernia

An *incisional hernia* occurs when an organ protrudes thru the incision line, for example, the intestines after an abdominal surgery. This is another risk, which may be caused by a patient's lifestyle or amount of mobility after the procedure. It is another complication that requires immediate attention because internal organs may be exposed and can cause necrosis. If any section of the intestine is without adequate blood supply, it can cause other complications, even death.

Multiple Surgeries

Each time a person has surgery, risks are present. The risks can increase or decrease depending on the procedure and type or route of the anesthetic. One surgical procedure may require additional procedures because of complications. If ample time is available, educate yourself prior to any procedure regarding the possibility for risks, additional procedures arising from complications, lifestyle, patient responsibility, and whether you are a good candidate for the procedure. Surgery requires an anesthetic each time a procedure is performed, and anesthetics also have risks. Prior to a procedure, do your homework to check if you are a candidate for the procedure in question and what your prognosis may be as influenced by your lifestyle.

Physicians

Medical personnel assist others to achieve or maintain a better quality of life. Communication between the medical staff and patient is critical for optimum care. If a patient withholds information that may allow better care—for example, about lifestyle and habits—then increased risks and complications may occur. Physicians may be able to diagnose and provide orders for treatment, but the patient must follow these orders to achieve the best possible prognosis. Patient responsibility is a very important piece to the healthcare puzzle, and if this is compromised, complications may occur, thereby reducing the quality of life. A physician can refuse to treat anyone if the patient's lifestyle is going to increase the risk for complications. Some patients represent a high risk for a surgeon. If the outcome will not satisfy the surgeon, and the risk outweighs the benefit, then the surgeon may not perform the procedure.

Preparation and preventative measures may be necessary to provide the best care possible.

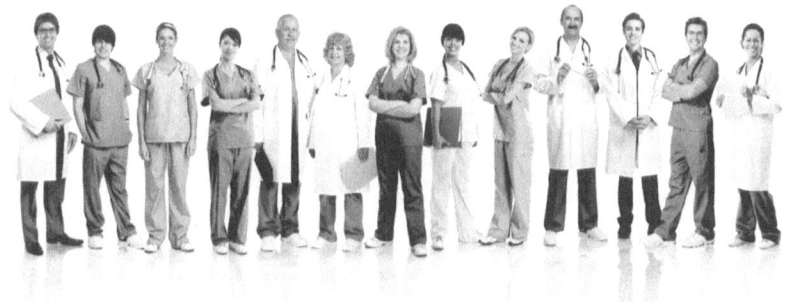

The more information the surgeon knows about you the better. All medical information is confidential, unless you allow in writing the release of information to specified persons.

Preoperative Instructions

Every patient receives instructions before and after any medical procedure, but it is the patient's responsibility to follow these orders for the best prognosis. Every patient is treated individually, even if the same surgical procedure is performed because of lifestyle. The instructions are provided prior to a procedure and include recommendations from the surgeon, facility, and the anesthesiologist. Prevention and preparation are the keys to lessening the risk of complications. These recommendations may begin as early as one year prior to the date of surgery—for example, the request to quit smoking. The surgeon may require a person seeking surgery to prepare prior to the procedure, and further prevention may be required as well for the best possible outcome.

Postoperative Instructions

The instructions given to a patient after a surgical procedure are very important. They may include information regarding mobility, bathing, prescriptions, wound care, durable medical equipment, home health care, and therapy. After the surgery, a nurse will instruct and provide the patient with a copy of the doctor's orders, contact number in case a problem occurs, and will explain that if a medical emergency arises, to call 911. It is a patient's responsibility to follow the orders given. The risk for complications increases for patients who do not do so. Lifestyle can determine a positive versus negative experience. The surgeon will assess the results from the procedure at a post-op appointment, unless a problem arises.

Patient Responsibility

Each patient has a responsibility to himself and to the medical personnel providing care. It is very important that each patient understands that lifestyle and habits can compromise a good prognosis. A surgeon may instruct a patient to refrain from nicotine, alcohol, or drug abuse for years, months, weeks, and even days before and/or after a procedure, and it is the patient's responsibility to follow the orders. A physician is seeking the best possible outcome for every patient, but sometimes this isn't possible because the patient will not follow the instructions.

Anatomy of the Female and Male

FEMALE

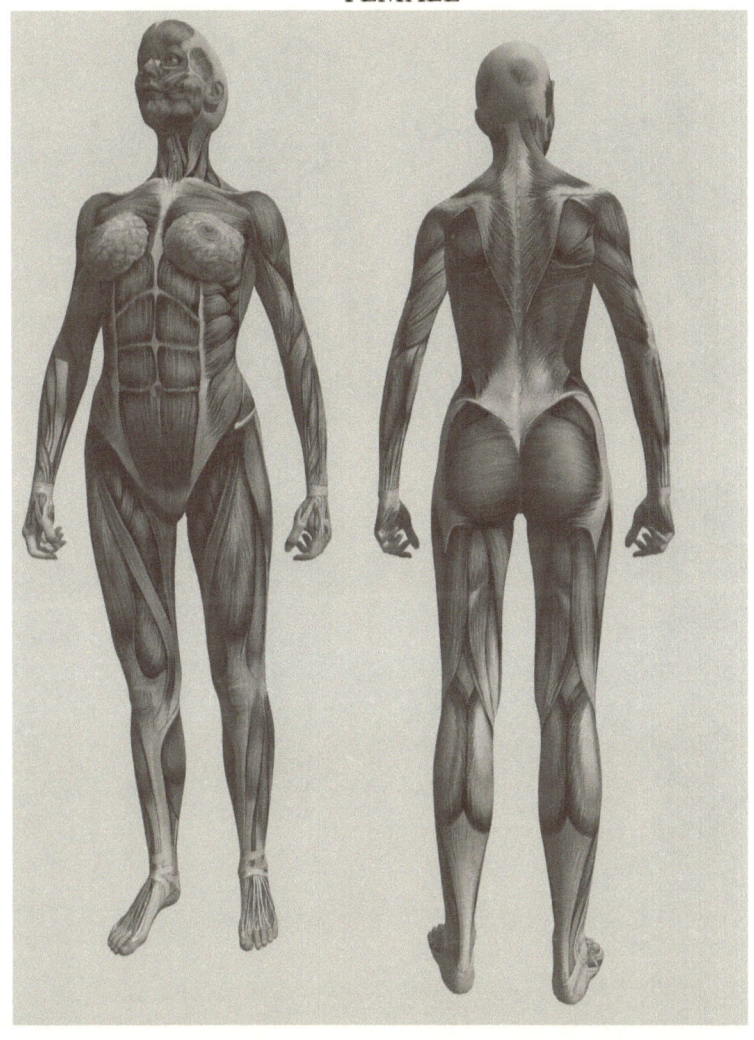

MALE

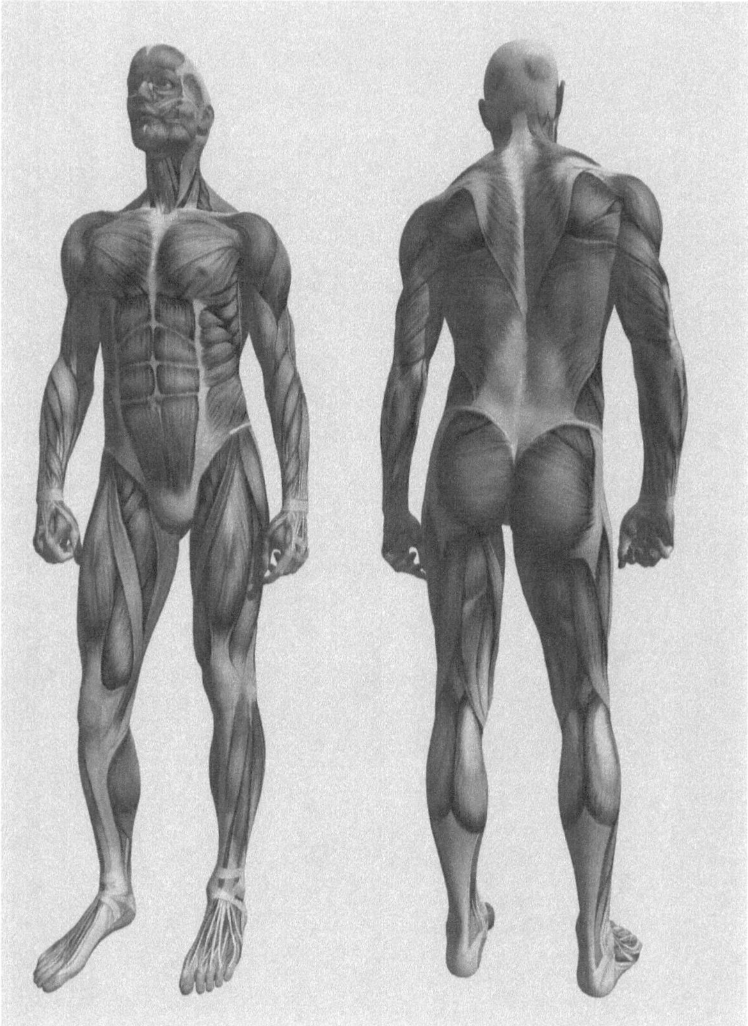

About the Author

Growing up, I was an active child. We lived in the country on a lake. I rode my bike all the time, and we always had a swimming pool. As soon as I reached puberty, I started to notice more fat appearing over my chest and stomach. Several years later, I noticed fat appearing on my upper arms. Over time, the fat increased all over my body, and I became less active. I was uncomfortable and lived with some kind of pain almost daily.

I have worked in health care most of my life and have observed firsthand the risks that being too fat can cause. I also watched my father suffer with heart disease caused by unhealthy nourishment choices, lack of consistent exercise, and smoking.

After many failed attempts to find a fast, easy way to lose fat, including fad diets and diet supplements, I contemplated surgery. Luckily, I have a low pain tolerance and chickened out every time. Because of the experiences I've had working in healthcare, I've seen the single surgery that turns into multiple surgeries because of scar tissue, further injury, or weight bearing on a particular muscle or joint, complications, infection, and so forth.

I noticed that many health care employees are fat and unhealthy just like me, and we were increasing our own risks of becoming the patient instead of the caregiver.

For years, I tried to incorporate healthy nourishment choices. I prepared meals at home daily and decreased the number of times that I went out to eat or consumed fast-food items. I had a multi-gym that I tried to use. Many years later I purchased a resort-size treadmill. For two years, I power walked three or more times a week and covered approximately five to ten miles a week. Because I was burning calories, I lost a couple of inches and some weight but still had fatty deposits. The more I worked out, the easier it became to make these changes, but I felt exhausted rather than energized after this type of workout. I remembered how I loved feeling strong when

I tried resistance training and I had the multi-station gym at my disposal, in addition to several free weights and dumbbells.

I realized that some of the foods I thought were healthy are not. What I needed was to lose fat, but most of what I was eating was high on the glycemic index! I finally learned about the glycemic index value and how it relates to the nourishment choices that we make every day.

During the course of five years of completed almost eighteen thousand pre-op surgery interviews for anesthesia at an orthopedic surgery center (approximately 4000 each year), I learned that most patients *are* uneducated about their own health.

I started a fitness and nutrition program that included proper nourishment choices daily to fuel my body and provide energy. It also included *"Black Jack" 21*, twenty-one resistance training exercises that will produce lean muscle mass and burn fat. This resistance is different for each individual and depends on the strength of the muscle or joint that is used.

This combination has stabilized my hormones, my mood, and my blood sugar levels, thereby decreasing my cravings and desire to binge. It has also decreased my aches and pains and has allowed me to lose the fatty deposits, decreasing my risk for health problems and increasing my life expectancy. In less than a year, I transformed my physique. The fat practically melted off and still is gone. I'm several sizes smaller than when I began and continue to show results every week. I am strong! I feel great! My hair, skin, nails, and teeth are in better health than ever before, and others tell me that I look ten years younger.

I encourage anyone who has ever tried to lose fat to take the *"Black Jack" to Lose Fat* challenge and get *your* body and groove back! And I commend anyone who can shake a weight for one minute, not to mention six minutes!

The year of 2011 has been the healthiest time of my life, and I attribute better health to the information provided in *"Black Jack" to Lose Fat, "Black Jack" to Get Your Health Back, and "Black Jack" to Prevent a Surgery Setback.* I suffered with chronic sinusitis for three years and the last year I couldn't taste or smell, so I procrastinated about having surgery for many reasons. I finally decided to have the surgery, but the symptoms soon returned. I was tired of being tired and sick of being sick.

These *"Black Jack"* guides include information regarding nourishment choices with real protein shakes made with Greek yogurt (no powders) and recipes that taste great; also the effects of poor health, medication, supplements, what we consume, have on the body, surgery risks, and two resistance training programs called *"Black Jack" 21* and *"Black Jack" 21 (Advanced Version)*, which I recommend that you perform three times a week. I have dealt with health problems most of my life, but since incorporating consistent resistance training and proper nourishment choices into my daily life, I feel great and no longer have to miss out on life because of being tired or sick.

Recipes and "Black Jack" Tips

Smoothies and Milk Shakes

Ice (unless the fruit is frozen)

Any type of milk or water

Greek yogurt (plain or vanilla)

Optional items include but aren't limited to: natural peanut butter/old fashioned peanut butter

cinnamon, vanilla, dark chocolate syrup, coffee, cayenne pepper

Fruit (any kind): blueberries, bananas, strawberries, peaches, mangos, mixed fruit, etc.

cayenne pepper speeds up the metabolism

"Black Jack" tip: Most fruits can be frozen. For example, peel bananas and place in Ziploc freezer bag.

Most fruits can also be found already frozen. Use within six months for optimum nutrient benefits.

(A blender is required.)

Chicken Curry

Cooked, deboned chicken, cut in chunks.
Place chicken in saucepan and one can of coconut milk; add curry to taste, and stir.
Optional items: frozen spinach or broccoli
Serve over Basmati rice.
Use more chicken than rice.
"Black Jack" tip: If trying to lose fat, always eat more protein than carbohydrates.

Peel and Eat Shrimp

Shrimp with shell on
Marinate in Italian dressing add tumeric, paprika, salt and pepper and garlic powder for fifteen minutes
 Sauté in EVOO and butter (Brummel & Brown yogurt butter) until pink or cooked thru
Peel Eat and Enjoy

Shrimp and Spinach

Shelled and deveined shrimp
Sauté in EVOO and butter until tender and/or pink (depending on type of shrimp), until the opaqueness is gone.
Add frozen spinach.
Serve over jasmine rice or your favorite pasta.
Use more shrimp and spinach than rice or pasta (try Seitenbacher all-natural pasta).
EVOO is extra virgin olive oil (try Pompeii Robust flavor).
"Black Jack" tip: Marinate shrimp in Italian salad dressing for ten minutes prior to cooking.

Pasta Salad

Deveined, shelled, and cooked shrimp or cooked, boneless, skinless chicken cubed
Cooked and chilled pasta
Vegetables
Italian salad dressing
Mix together; serve cold.
Any vegetables, such as cucumbers, broccoli, scallions, tomatoes, peppers, carrots, celery, mushrooms, or onions
Optional items: cheese, olives
Broccoli can be slightly cooked or blanched.

Quesadillas

Tortillas, any kind, any size
Deveined and peeled shrimp, lean chicken, beef, pork, or fish
Cook shrimp, fish, or meat in frying pan with EVOO and butter.
Add garlic, onions, or other vegetables and spices.
Optional items: cheese, rice, sour cream, guacamole, olives, beans
Place tortilla in frying pan, add preferred fillings, and top with another tortilla.
Heat on low until warm; flip and warm other side until cheese melts tortillas together.
Top with optional items

Experiment with Food and Spices

I learned to cook with my Italian grandmother Yia-Yia and my father who was Greek and Italian neither one of them ever measured anything. This is how I know Cooking is not rocket science, and it can be great fun and a master craft to improving your health.

Cooking at home allows you to know exactly what is in your food—if you are trying to lose fat, then you don't need hidden fats and calories that hide in food you do not prepare, and it saves a ton of money.

"Black Jack" tips: If you have prepared foods available all the time and don't allow yourself to become hungry,

fast food can become part of the past.

Cinnamon Toast

Bread
Butter
Cinnamon
Sugar
Butter bread, sprinkle with cinnamon sugar, and toast, broil, or bake until butter melts and bread is a little crunchy.

Cheese Toast

Bread
Cheese
Top bread with cheese or cheeses and toast, broil, or bake until cheese is melted and bread is a little crunchy.
Optional items: basil and tomatoes

Poached Eggs

Bread (toasted)
Poached eggs
Poach eggs and place over bread (toasted).
Optional: cheese on bread prior to toasting
Eggs can be poached in boiling water, and egg poacher trays are available.
Include fats, carbohydrates, and proteins with every meal or snack.
"Black Jack" tip: It's great to hard-boil eggs ahead of time and grab them as needed.

Scrambled Eggs

Scramble eggs and cook in pan with butter
Optional items: cheese, frozen spinach thawed, asparagus, onion, green yellow or red peppers
"Black Jack" tip: make a large amount and place in a crust or pan and bake in oven 350 degrees until firm and fully cooked

Egg Sandwich

Fry egg and place on bread or toast; add mayonnaise and/or cheese.

Too Awesome Soup

In saucepan, simmer on low a few tablespoons of EVOO, butter, and chopped garlic;
do not burn the garlic, or the soup will be bitter.
Add two to four quarts of tomato juice and stir.
Add fresh-squeezed lemon, optional pepper to taste, cayenne pepper or hot sauce, and stir.
Add vegetables cut up in chunks, such as fresh eggplant, zucchini, squash, peppers, onions, or mushrooms;
leave skin on the vegetables.
Bring to a boil, and then simmer until vegetables are tender (usually about an hour).
Cooking time will vary depending on the size of your vegetable chunks.
"Black Jack" tip: Add mushrooms about thirty minutes before serving.
Add a tablespoon of sugar per two quarts.
"Black Jack" tip: Sugar cuts down the acidity of tomato products and lowers the risk of indigestion and heartburn,
especially in tomato sauces.

Pears or Apples and Cheese or Old-Fashioned Peanut Butter

Pears
Apples
Cheeses or old-fashioned or natural peanut butter
A balanced snack and an excellent pick-me-up to fuel the body for the next half of the day.

Unsweetened Applesauce and Cottage Cheese

One part unsweetened applesauce
One part cottage cheese
Mix together.

It's an awesome snack.

Spicy Nuts

Any kind of shelled nuts; separate or mix them together.
Try Seitenbacher nuts (all natural).
Heat olive oil and butter in a pan over low heat; add nuts and stir.
Spread nuts on baking sheet and sprinkle with spices.
Optional spices:
Five spice
Garlic powder
Curry
Cinnamon
Sugar
Wasabi
Mrs. Dash products
Turmeric
Paprika
"Black Jack" tip: You control the amount of spices.
These are a great snack, appetizer, and gift (include the recipe).

Avocado

Peel and slice or slice and eat right out of the skin, topped with salt and pepper.
"Black Jack" tip: An avocado is best when still a little firm but tender to the touch.
If shaken, you can hear and feel the seed moving

Avocado Milkshake (contains coffee)

Ice
Avocado
Espresso or coffee
Sweetened condensed milk or any kind of milk
Vanilla
Blend together.
Optional: line cup with dark chocolate syrup
Top with whipped cream and dark chocolate syrup.

Tomato and Cheese

Bread, slightly buttered (on the outside of the bread)
Sliced tomato
Cheese
Grill each side of this sandwich in a frying pan over low heat.

Tomato Sandwich

Bread
Tomato (sliced)
Mayonnaise (regular)
Salt and pepper

Wraps

Tortillas, any kind and size
Filling options:
Beans
Rice
Cooked fish, shrimp, lean meats, or poultry
Warm up the filling, place in wrap, and roll.
"Black Jack" tip: Mix together sour cream and drained black beans and spread on tortillas.
Wrap, chill, and cut into slices.
Serve cold.
A great appetizer or snack.

PB&J

Bread

Old-fashioned or natural peanut butter
Simply Fruit spread
Serve with a glass of milk.

Hummus

one cup ground garbanzo beans or chickpeas
one tablespoon EVOO
Juice from one half of a lemon
Optional items: chopped, sundried tomatoes, olives, crushed red pepper flakes
Serve with cracker or pita chips.

Cream Cheese and Jelly or Salsa

Cream cheese and salsa or red pepper, jalapeno, peach, pear jelly, etc.
Serve with crackers.

Notes

Notes

Notes

Notes

Notes

Notes